COOKIE DOUGHGA

A Book about yoga, mindfulness, and cookies!

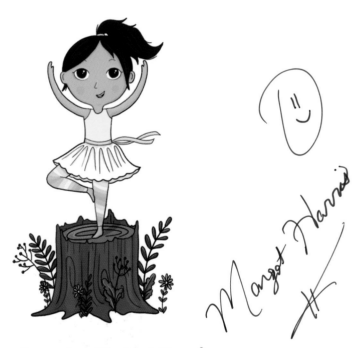

Written by: Margot Harris
Illustrated by: Stefanie Geyer

For my Mama

Love,

your "Cookie girl"

Cookie Doughga
A book about yoga, mindfulness, and cookies!

Copyright © 2020 Margot Harris

ISBN: 978-1-09834-229-6

Library of Congress Control Number: 2020918216

Names, characters, and places are products of the author's imagination.

Front cover image, illustrations, and book design by Stefanie Geyer.

First printing edition 2020.

Signature Book Printing
www.sbpbooks.com

Visit the authors website:
www.calmcookie.org
to schedule an event, host classes or workshops, or to request persmissions.

To connect on social media, join Margot's Instagram community @calmcookie_kidsyoga.

Dear grown ups,

Thank you for buying this book! I hope it brings you as much joy as it has brought me.

The kids in your life will always need you for guidance, encouragement, and above all—love. They also need to believe in themselves! Yoga and mindfulness practices can be a fun way to teach children to explore their inner voice, resources, and power. Learning to connect to their thoughts, feelings, and body shows them that they have the ability to face any challenge. When big feelings arise, kids don't always know how to cope or even what to call them. This book offers simple mindfulness techniques that can help children notice and deal with their feelings.

The yoga poses in this book will provide children a chance to move mindfully and become aware of how it makes their body feel. For example, mountain, tree, and warrior are good for grounding and connection when they are feeling anxious or scattered. Airplane, frog, and triangle might give your child a boost in energy. Cobra, cat, and downward dog are playful and engage your child's natural joy and wonder. Child's pose can provide a sense of comfort and relaxation.

You can teach your child to be an explorer of their mind and body. Yoga creates space for self awareness, growth, and curiosity about their experiences. Remember to let them know that it's OK to stop if something doesn't feel right for their body at any given time.

Most importantly, be present and have fun!

Peace & Love & Cookies,
Margot

1

Maria and her Mama made some cookie dough.

Air was sweet, filled with heat. The sun was setting low.

"What to do with all this dough?" wondered Mama aloud.

"Cookies doing yoga!" squealed Maria, feeling proud.

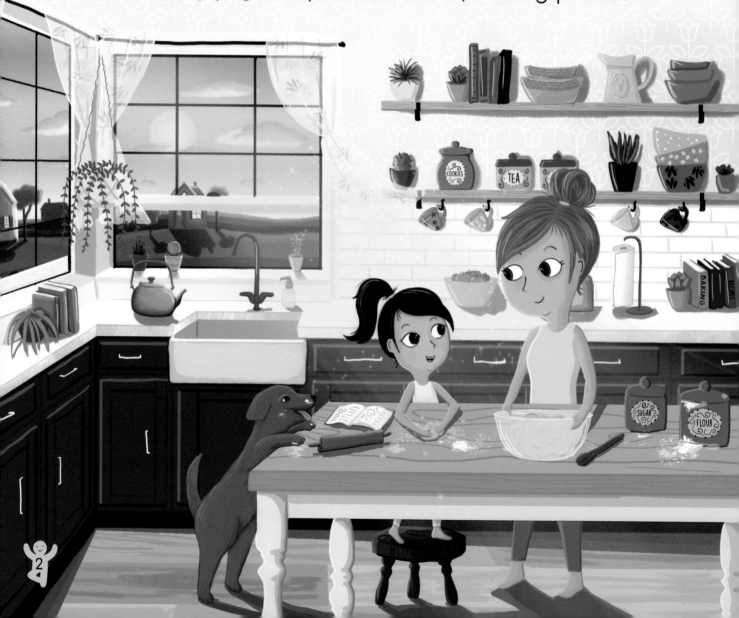

They rolled, and kneaded, and twisted, and turned.
They patted, and flattened, and molded, and churned.
When they were finished they looked upon
all of the hard work they had done.

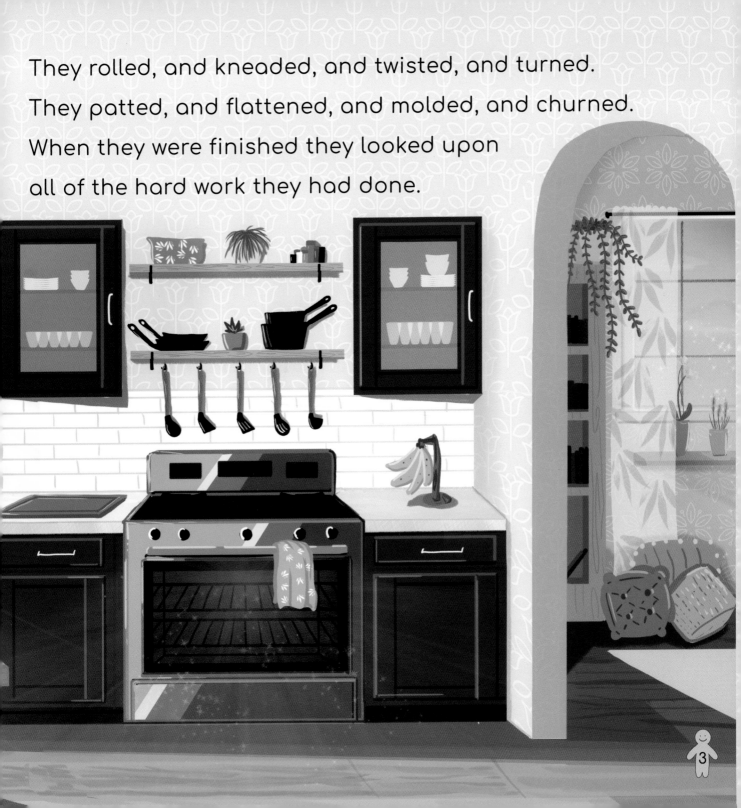

Maria's dough now looked like yoga.

She giggled and called it "cookie doughga."

Mama chuckled, "The oven's hot!

Let's pop them in and set the clock."

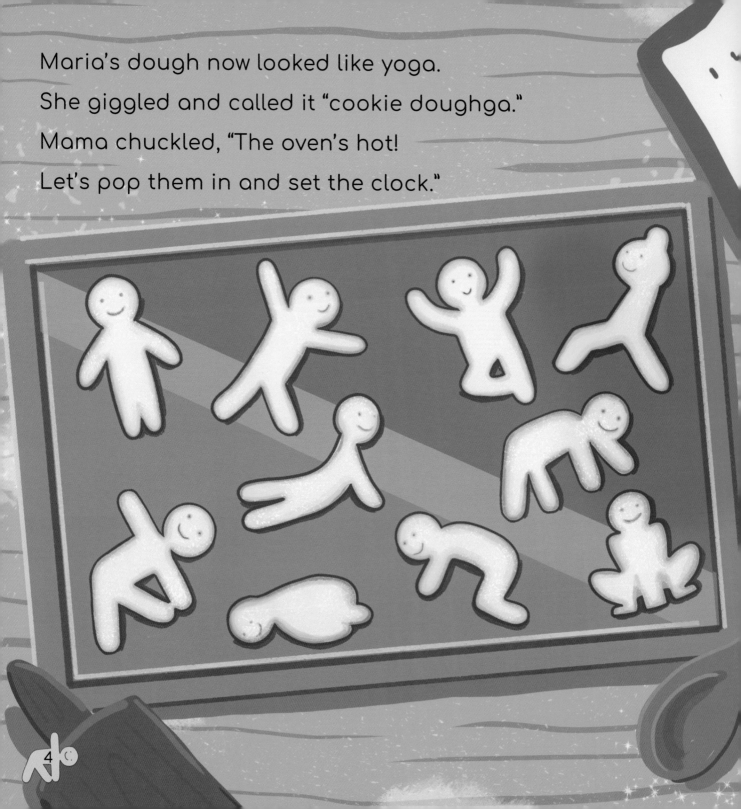

"While we wait, let's have some fun.
We'll practice yoga 'til they're done."
Mama beamed, "Another great idea!
Let's get moving, my sweet Maria."

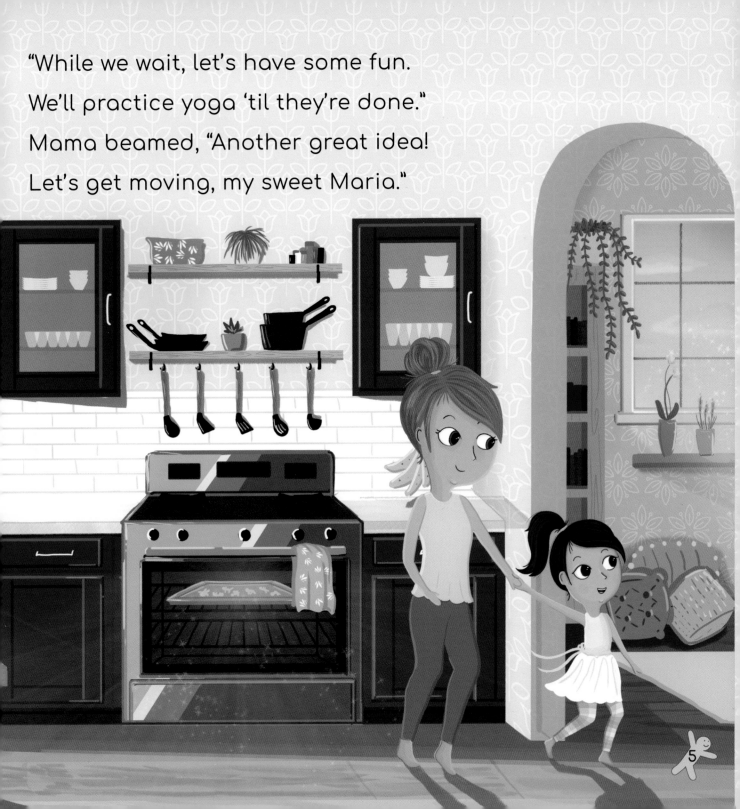

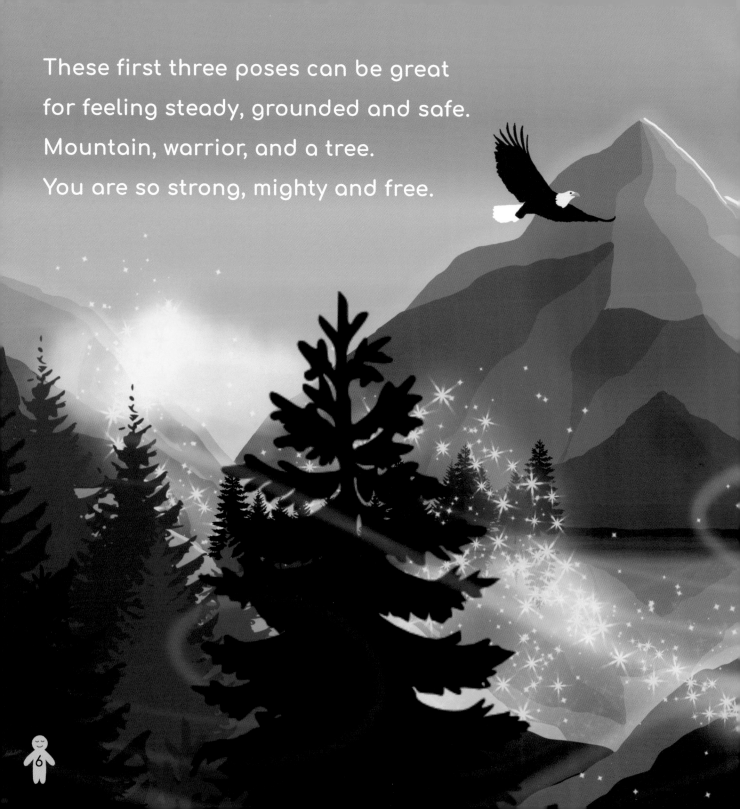

These first three poses can be great
for feeling steady, grounded and safe.
Mountain, warrior, and a tree.
You are so strong, mighty and free.

Mountain pose

Like a mountain, be steady and tall.

Wild winds can't make your body fall!

Stand up straight with both feet flat.

How does your body feel like that?

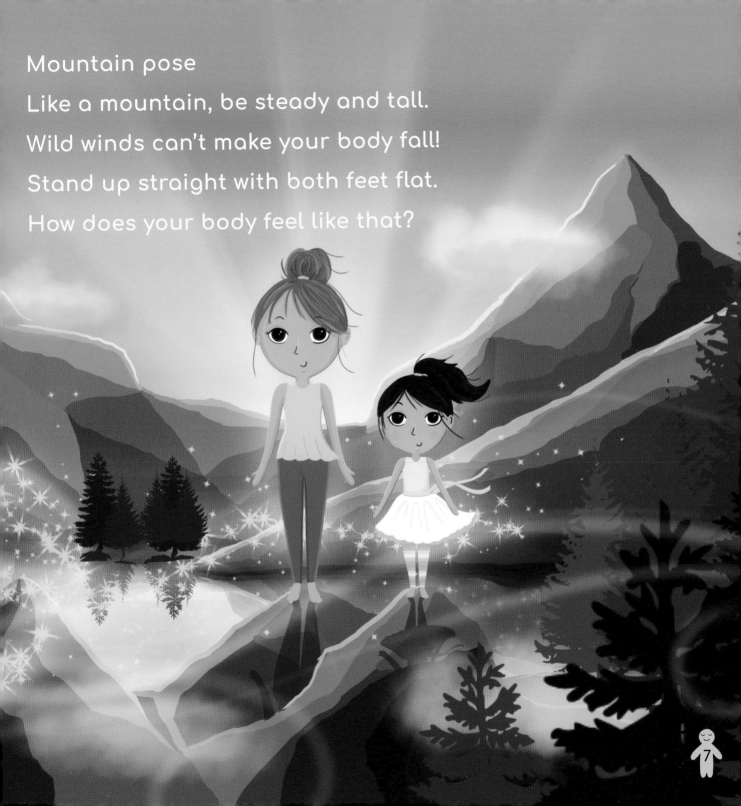

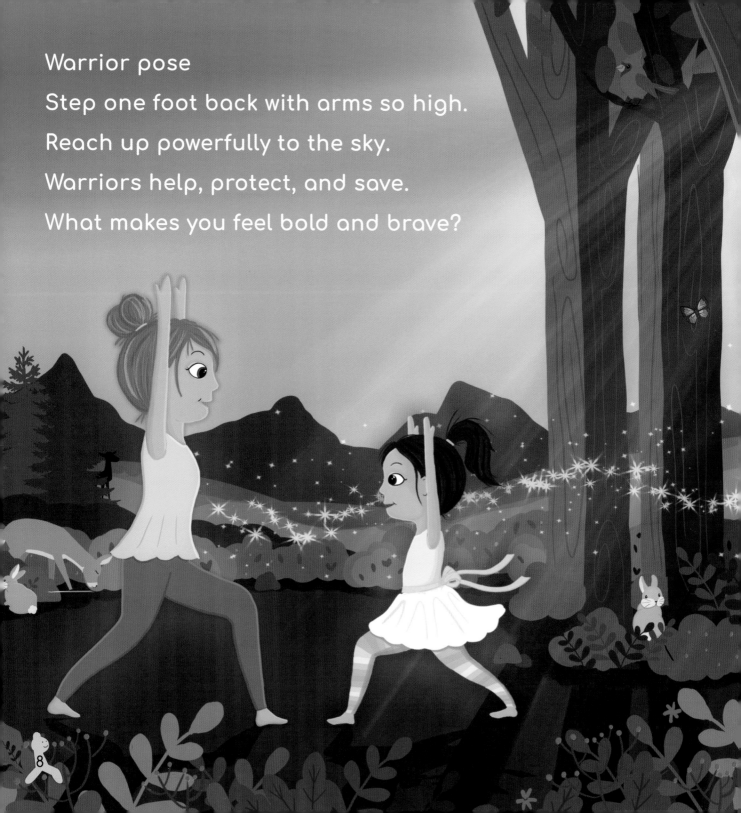

Warrior pose

Step one foot back with arms so high.

Reach up powerfully to the sky.

Warriors help, protect, and save.

What makes you feel bold and brave?

Tree pose

Plant one foot and bend your knee.

Now you are a special tree!

Your roots are deep, your branches long.

Can you hold your body strong?

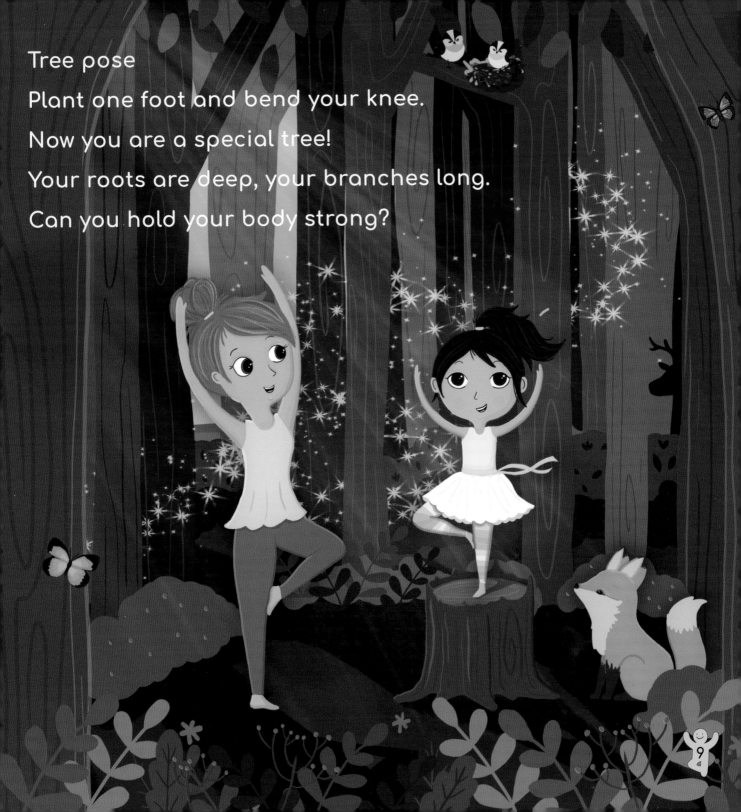

These next three poses might just be
the ones to give you energy.
When you balance, jump, and bend
your mind and body are best friends.

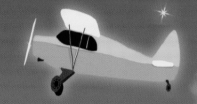

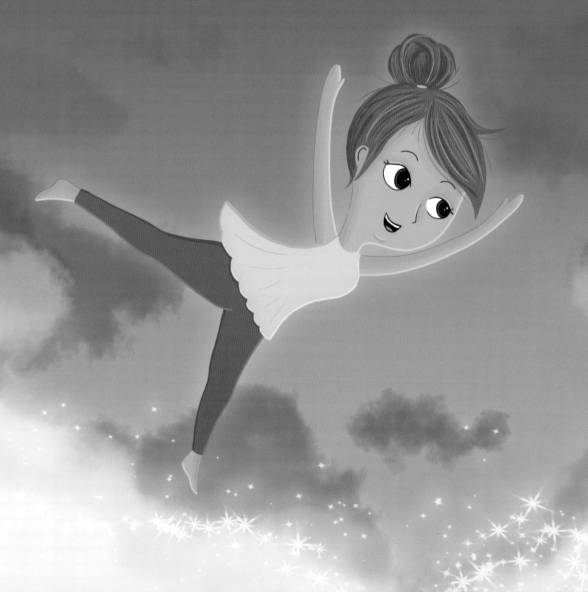

Airplane pose

Stretch one leg back, it's time to fly.

Bring your wings out to the side.

Lift your back leg off the floor.

Who or what makes your heart soar?

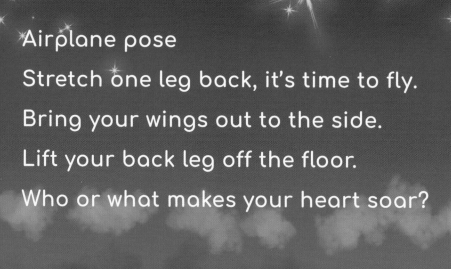
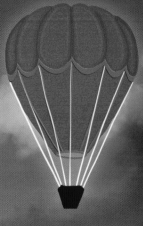
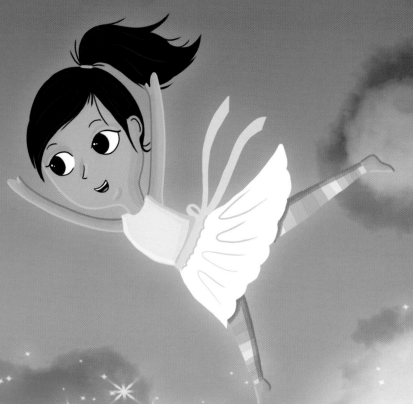

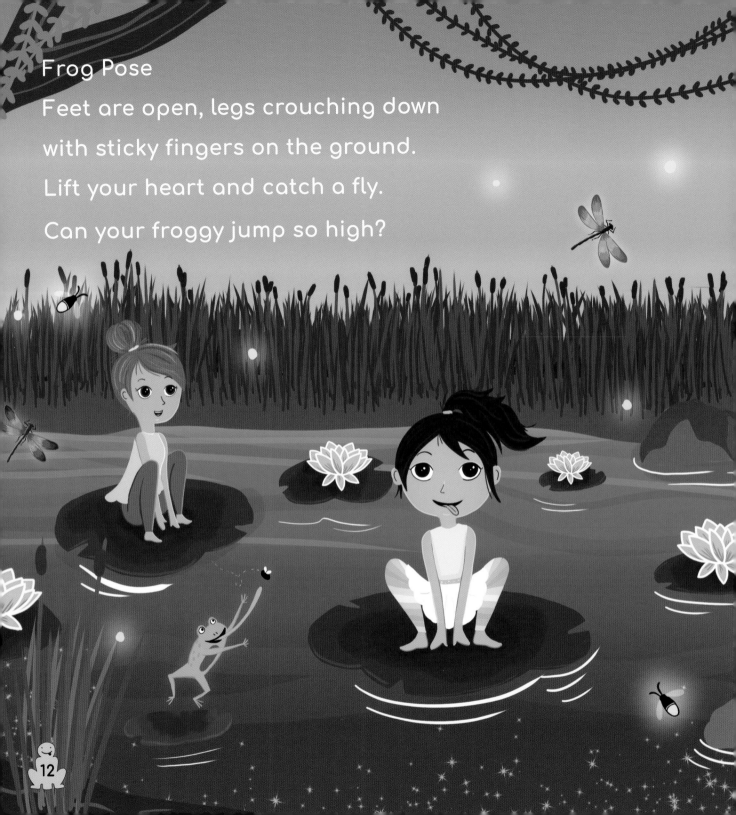

Frog Pose

Feet are open, legs crouching down
with sticky fingers on the ground.
Lift your heart and catch a fly.
Can your froggy jump so high?

12

Triangle pose

Jump your feet apart so wide.

Point one foot out to the side.

Spread your arms and lean down low.

Can you touch your little toes?

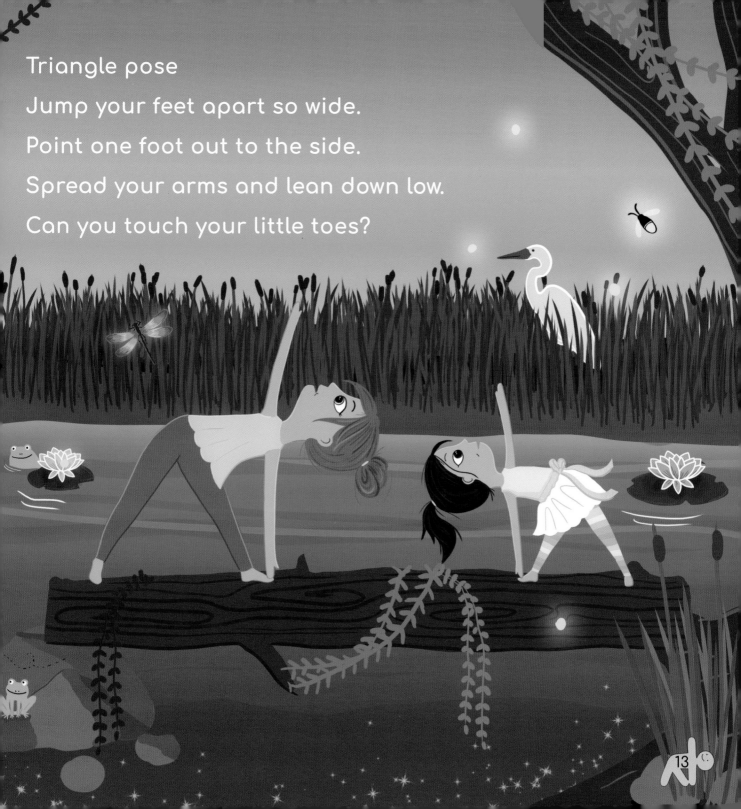

These three poses stretch the spine.

Open your heart and let it shine!

Cobra, cat, and downward dog

can ease the mind and clear the fog.

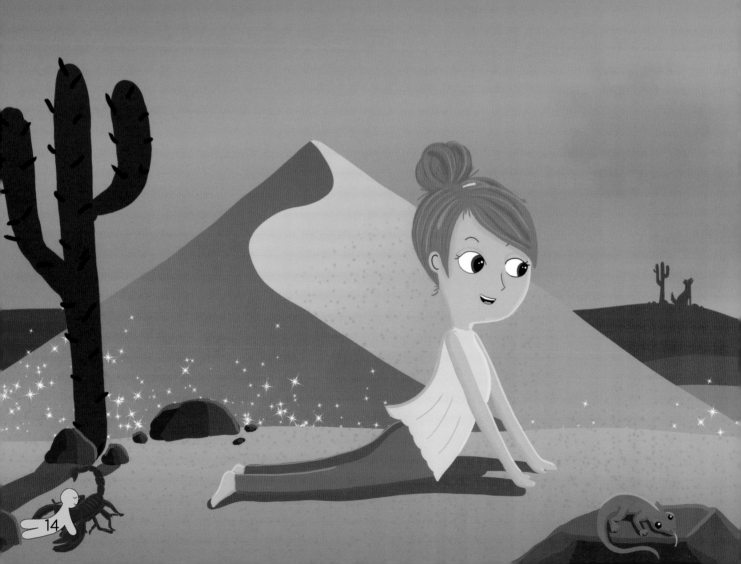

Cobra Pose

Bring your belly to the sand.

Lift your heart up off the land.

Breathe in and hiss, look side to side.

Can your cobra slither and slide?

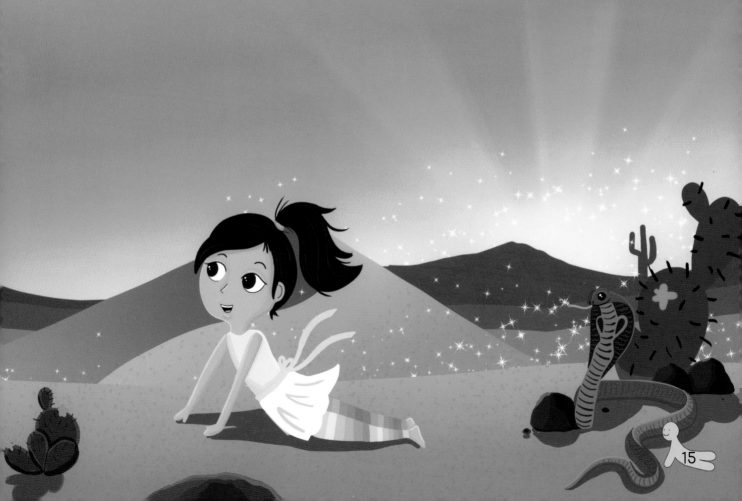

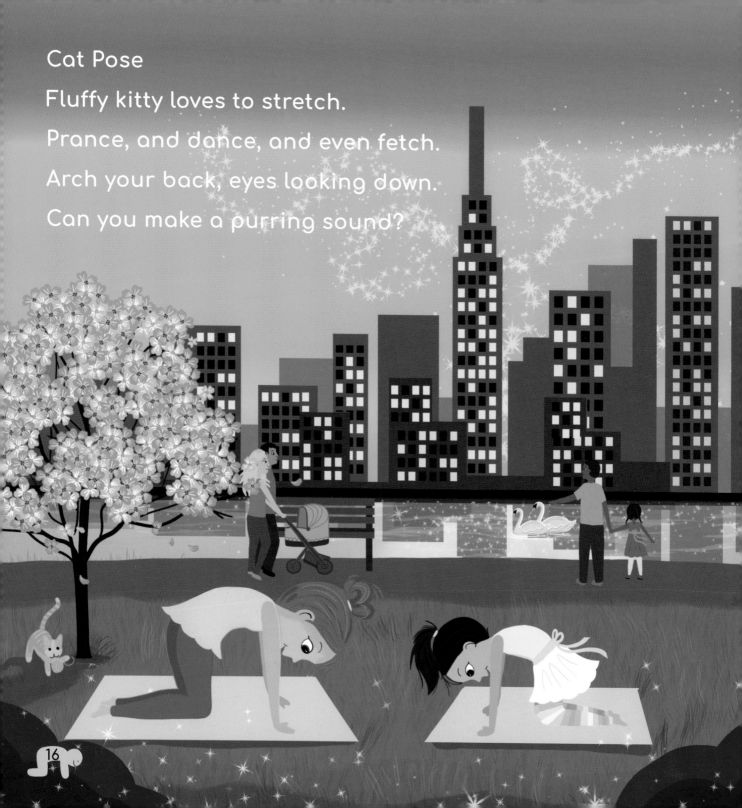

Cat Pose

Fluffy kitty loves to stretch.

Prance, and dance, and even fetch.

Arch your back, eyes looking down.

Can you make a purring sound?

16

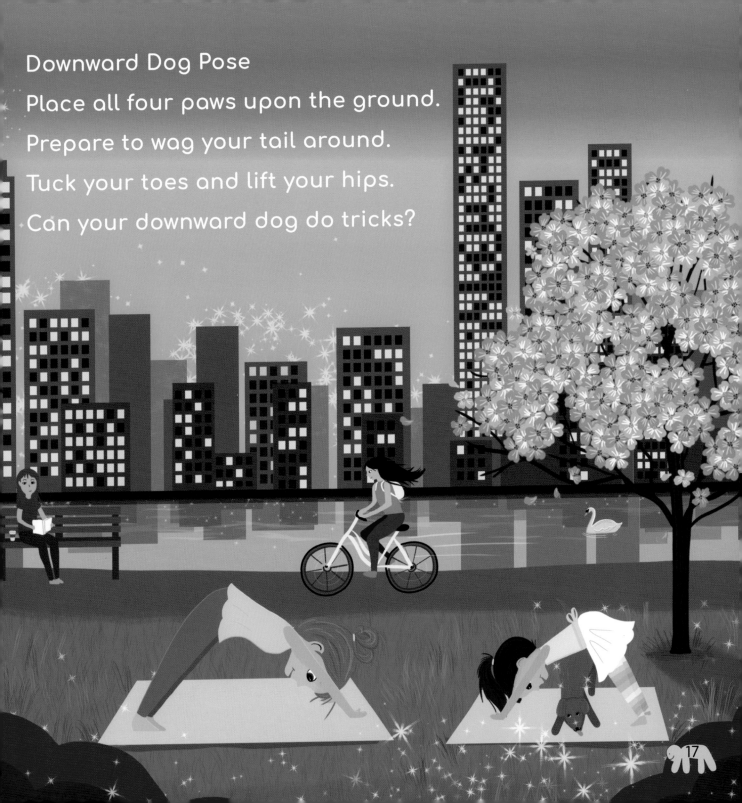

Downward Dog Pose

Place all four paws upon the ground.

Prepare to wag your tail around.

Tuck your toes and lift your hips.

Can your downward dog do tricks?

17

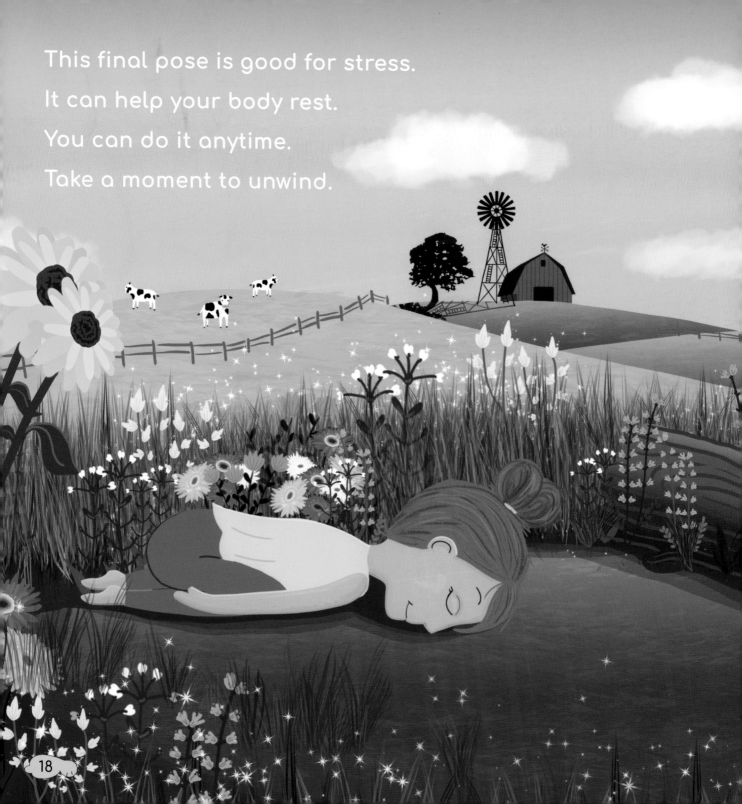

This final pose is good for stress.

It can help your body rest.

You can do it anytime.

Take a moment to unwind.

Child's pose

Curl up like a little mouse,
dozing and dreaming in a house.
Say this mantra in your mind:
"I am peaceful, brave, and kind."

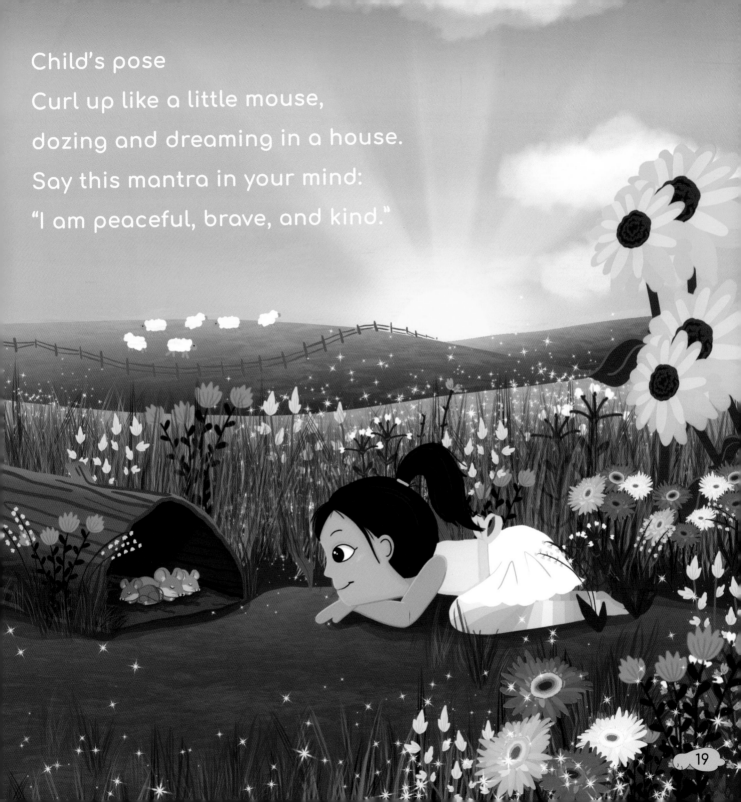

Suddenly the oven beeped, the cookies almost done.
"One minute left!" Maria cried, as she began to run.
Mama laughed and nodded as Maria zoomed by.
"Practicing yoga seemed to make time fly!"

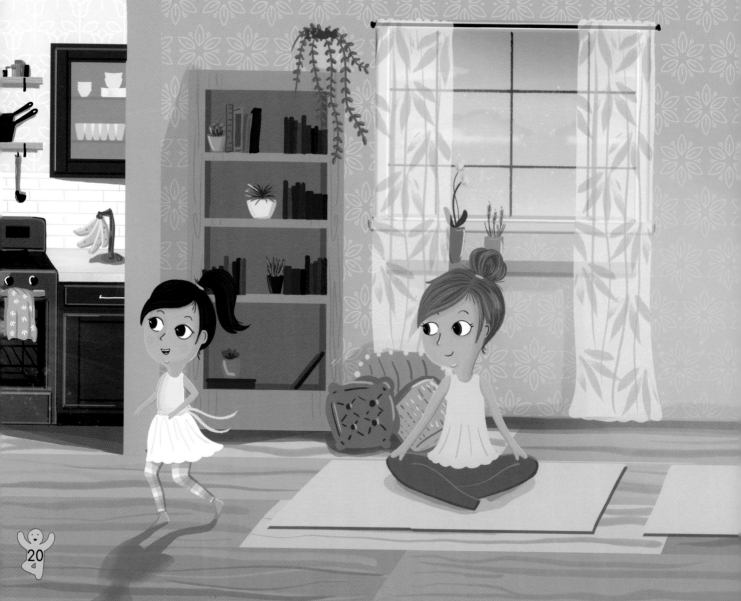

As Maria continued to wait,

her mind began to contemplate.

"What if the cookies aren't good enough?

What if they're too burnt or too tough?"

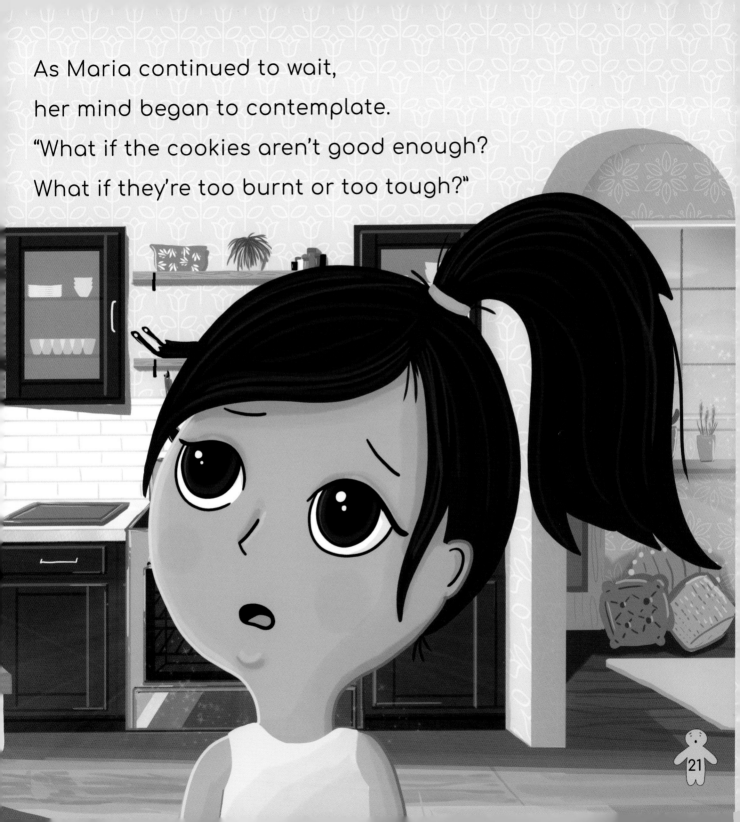

"Oh my sweet Maria girl,
it's normal for your thoughts to twirl.
When big feelings circle and spin,
connect to your body and check in."

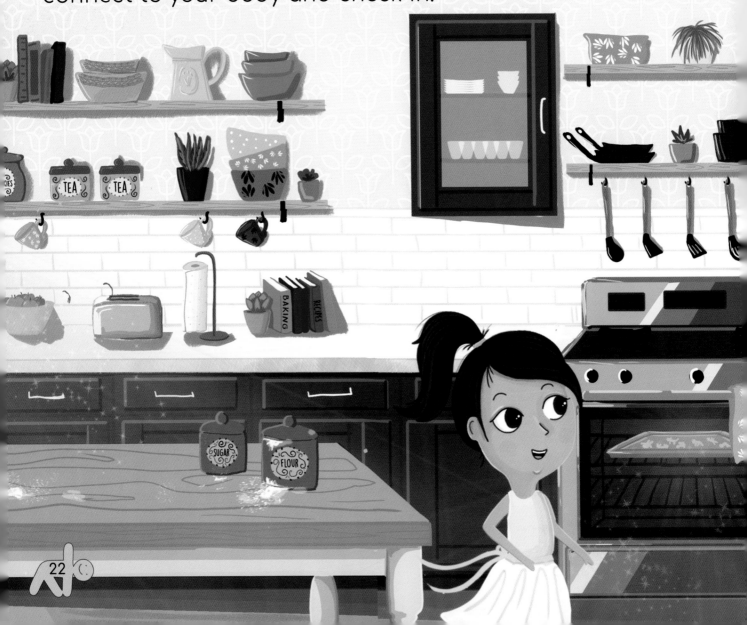

"That's true," Maria raised her voice.
"How I feel can be a choice.
I have the tools inside of me
to send my worries out to sea."

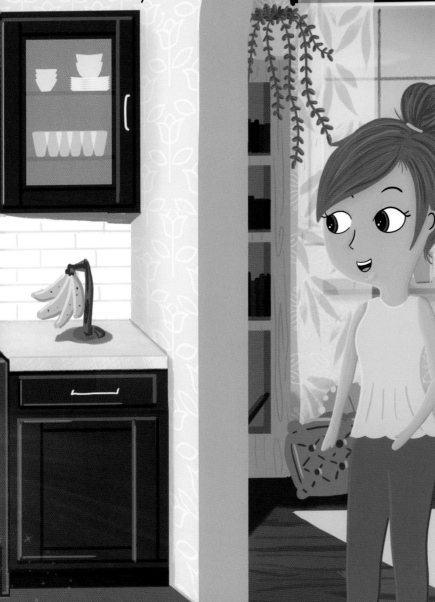
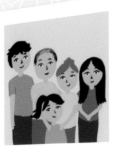
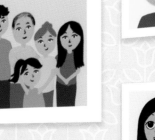
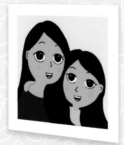

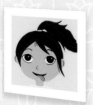

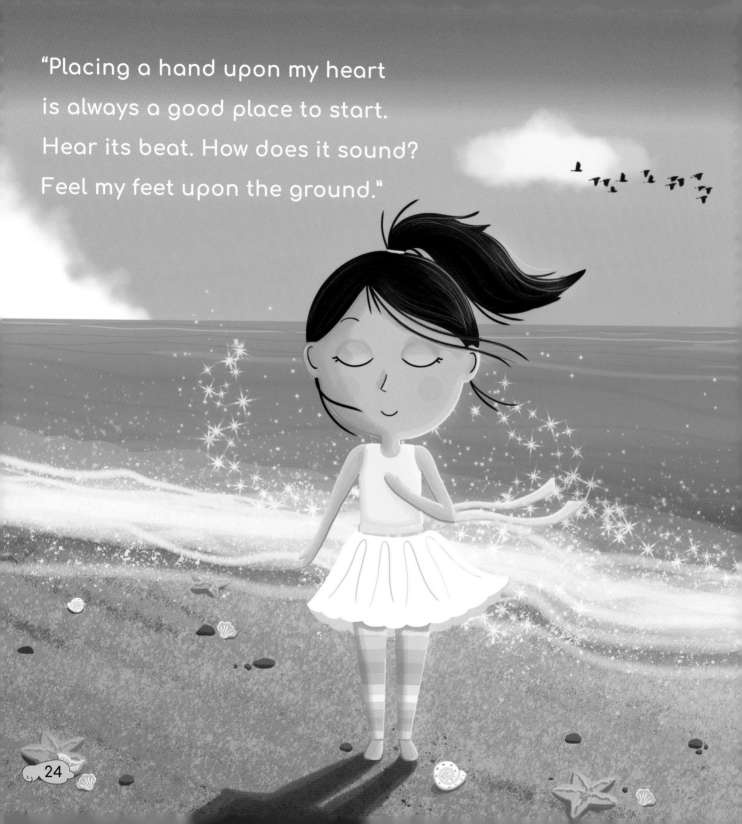

"Placing a hand upon my heart
is always a good place to start.
Hear its beat. How does it sound?
Feel my feet upon the ground."

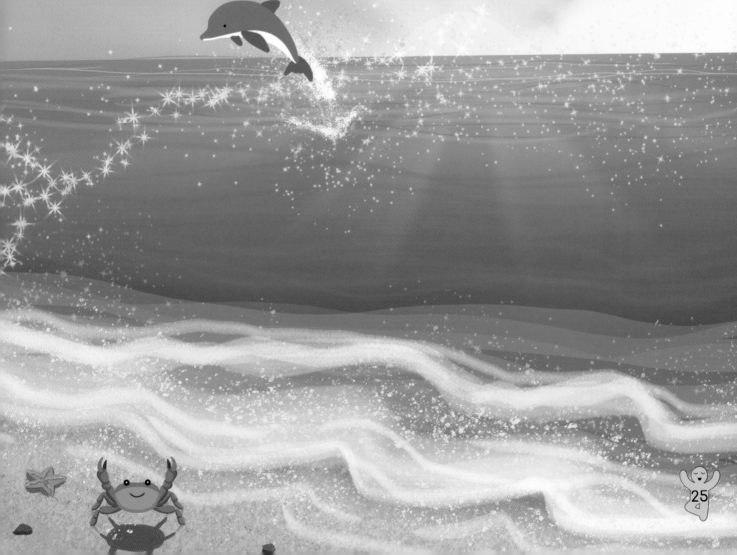

"Take three deep and steady breaths.
Pause for a moment and reflect.
I had oodles of fun today,
baking cookies in my own new way!"

Maria cheered, "I feel alright!
I'm proud of what I've done tonight.
Stretching, and changing, like the dough.
I'll keep learning as I grow."

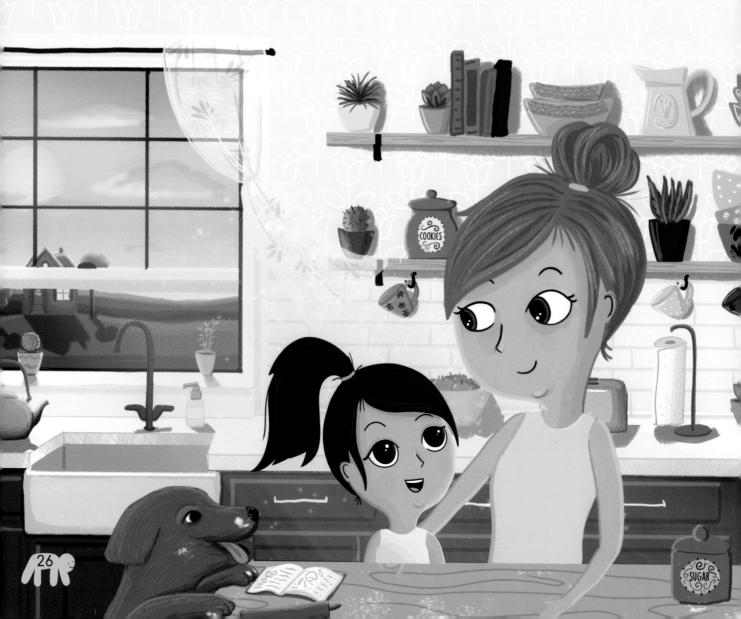

26

"Cookies come and cookies go.
No matter what, I'll always know—
I can trust myself to see
all the good inside of me."

Ding.

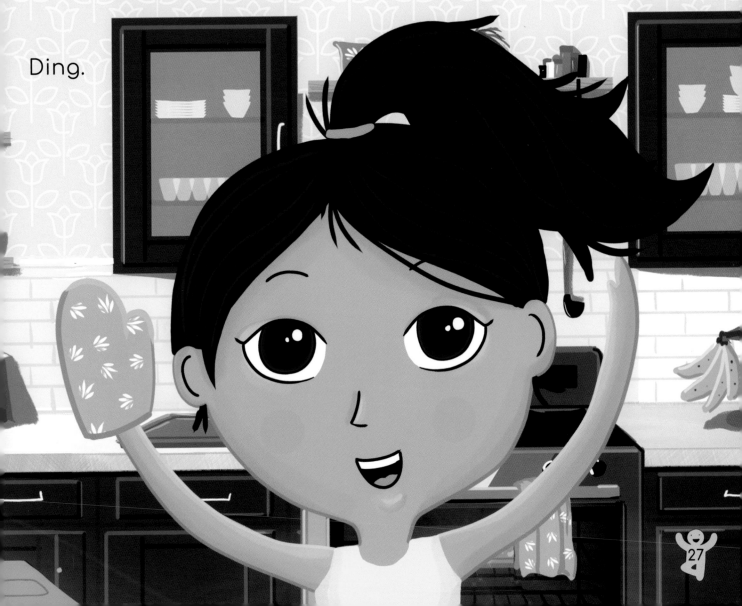

Simple Sugar Cookies

This simply sweet sugar cookie recipe is perfect for making your very own Cookie Doughga! Use cookie cutters, or have fun creating the shapes yourself. Add your own flair by accessorizing with decorations like sprinkles, cinnamon sugar, royal icing, or even chocolate chips!

Ingredients:
3/4 cups butter, softened (1 1/2 sticks)
1 cup white sugar
2 eggs
1/2 teaspoon vanilla extract
2 1/2 cups all-purpose flour
1 teaspoon baking powder
1/2 teaspoon salt

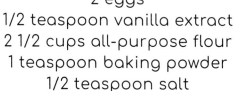

Directions:
1. In a large bowl, blend together butter and sugar until smooth. Beat in eggs and vanilla. Stir in the flour, baking powder, and salt. Mix well until thoroughly combined. Cover and chill dough for at least 1 hour (or overnight).

2.Preheat the oven to 400 degrees F (200 degrees C). Roll out dough on a floured surface 1/4 to 1/2 inch thick. Cut into shapes with any cookie cutter OR get creative with making your own shapes. Place cookies 1 inch apart on ungreased cookie sheets.

3.Bake 6-8 minutes in the preheated oven. Time will vary depending on size and shape of the cookies and your oven type.

4.Cool completely, and enjoy!

***Recipe yields approximately 25-50 cookies, largely depending on size and shape, use of cookie cutters or not.
***Recommend adding decorations after baking is complete.

Acknowledgements

Adam- My love, my constant. You heard every draft of this story, and gave me fresh eyes and perspective at every step. Your laid back nature and go with the flow attitude is the yin to my yang. I continue to be in awe of your talent, your generosity, your warm and tender heart. Even after 20 years, you continue to amaze and surprise me. There is no one I'd rather share my everything with. There will never be enough words of gratitude. I love you.

Mom and Dad- You are my very foundation, the ground upon which I stand. Your relentless love and support has always made me feel safe and capable. Whenever my anxiety took over as I grew, I knew I could always count on you to be there. You never rushed me, but encouraged me with kindness, empathy, laughter, and joy. You were my first mindfulness teachers. Thank you, thank you, thank you. I love you.

Lisa and Pete- My big sister and brother. From you both, I've learned so much about exploring passions, setting big goals and dreams, and raising the bar. You inspire me to keep pushing, keep learning, and that there's always another opportunity to be had. Your fierce love and support through my entire life has been beyond what a little sister could hope for. I love you.

Betty- I very literally could not have done this without you. Your wisdom, kindness, and openness helped make this story everything I could've wanted it to be. Thank you for sharing your expertise, guidance, and firm belief with me. You helped find mine and Maria's voice. I'll always be grateful.

Stefanie- Your art has brought my words to life. Its whimsy and unique character bring instant smiles to my face, and I know it will do the same for many others. I'm so thankful that you agreed to work with me. You made every step of the process not just easy, but fun! I can't wait to collaborate with you again in the future.

Friends and colleagues- Your support and love mean the world. Thank you for your feedback, encouragement, and belief in me always. I love you.

To all my students- Past, Present, and Future. You inspire me daily. You are the reason I do this work. You are incredible humans. You are capable. You are beautiful. You matter. I'm honored to know you. I love you.

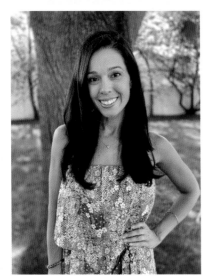

Margot Harris is a children's yoga and mindfulness educator from Long Island, NY. Her goal is to empower children to trust themselves, and believe in the strength of their bodies, minds and hearts. She loves to dance, go to the movies, and listen to the ocean. Taking long neighborhood walks with her husband Adam and their dog Hurley after a long day brings peace to her heart. Laughing with family, and friends is her most favorite thing to do. That, and eating all the cookies!

Stefanie Geyer is a children's book illustrator from Winamac, Indiana. She works in many medias such as digital, pencil, and paint. In her spare time she enjoys drawing portraits of people and animals. Speaking of animals, Stefanie is an avid animal lover. She lives with her boyfriend Chris and their five dogs Halen, Presley, Kimber, Roux, and Draco! She loves nature, a good hike in the woods, gardening, and home renovation projects.

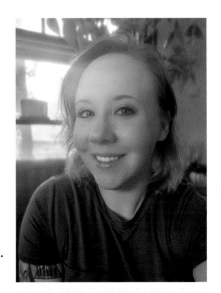